ALLERGIES

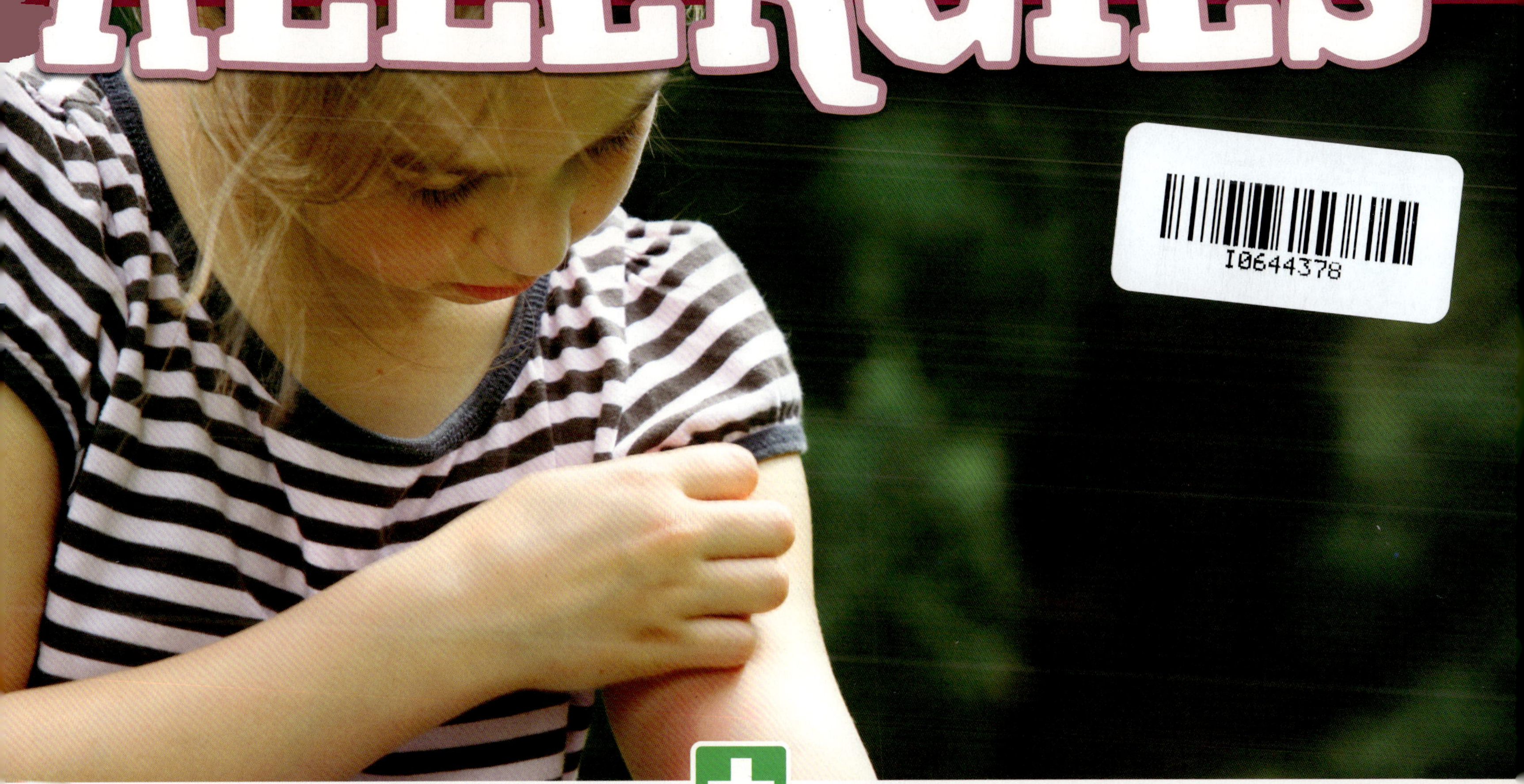

IN CASE OF EMERGENCY

Helen Lepp Friesen
and Ryan Smith

AV2
www.av2books.com

Step 1
Go to **www.av2books.com**

Step 2
Enter this unique code

QHMVDJAS0

Step 3
Explore your interactive eBook!

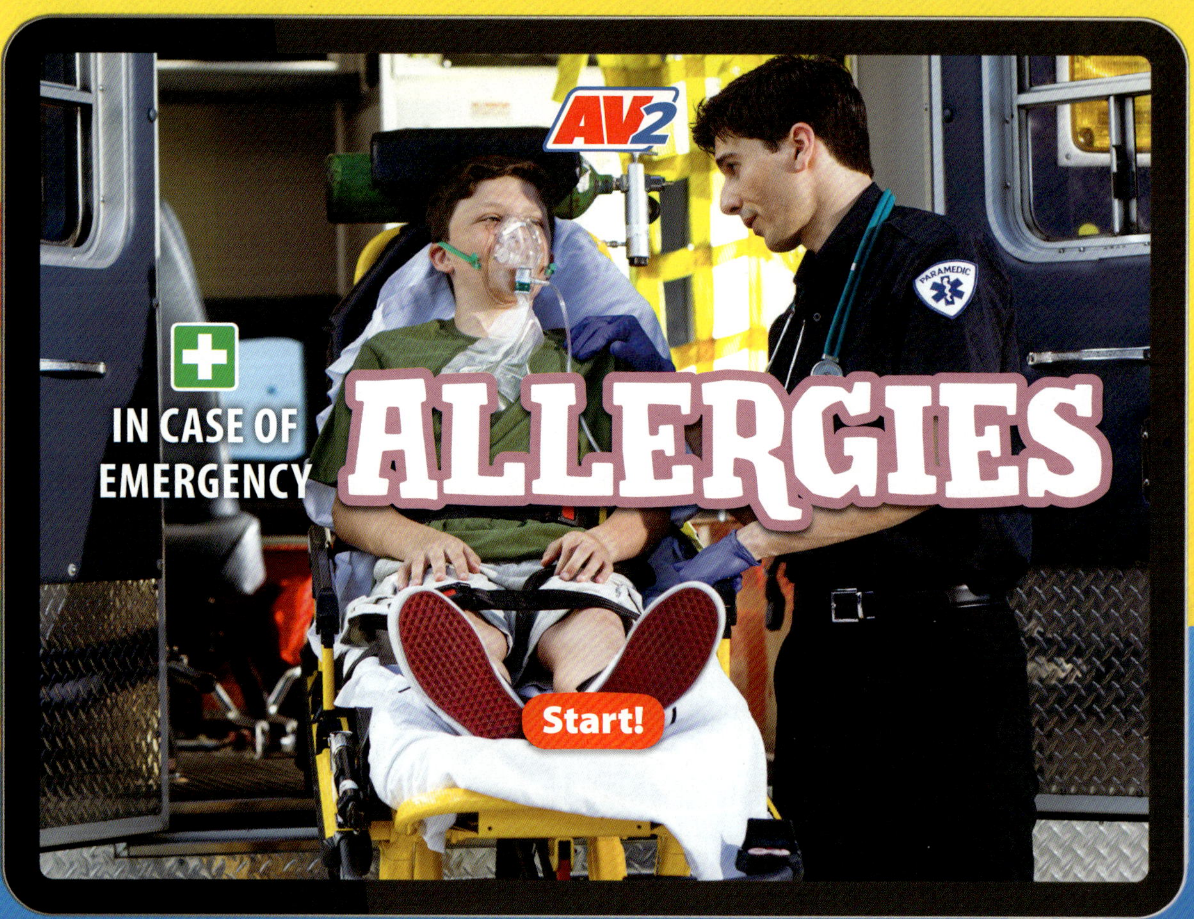

AV2 is optimized for use on any device

Your interactive eBook comes with...

Read

- **Audio** Listen to the entire book read aloud
- **Videos** Watch informative video clips
- **Weblinks** Gain additional information for research
- **Try This!** Complete activities and hands-on experiments
- **Key Words** Study vocabulary, and complete a matching word activity
- **Quizzes** Test your knowledge
- **Slideshows** View images and captions

View new titles and product videos at www.av2books.com

IN CASE OF EMERGENCY

ALLERGIES

Contents

2 AV2 Book Code
4 The Emergency: An Allergic Reaction
6 Signs and Symptoms
8 Stay Calm
10 Call 9-1-1
12 Rescue Step 1: Move Away
14 Rescue Step 2: Give Medicine
16 Rescue Step 3: Rest
18 Help Arrives
20 Preventative Measures
22 Emergency Procedures
24 Key Words

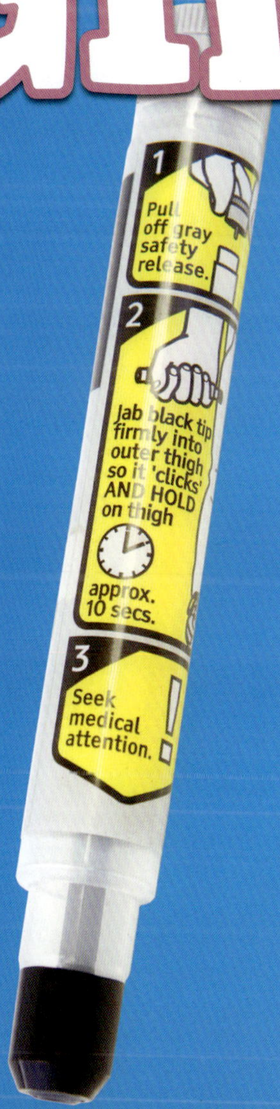

An Allergic Reaction

Some people have allergies to food, insects, plants, dust, or medicines.

A small reaction can make a person feel itchy.

A big reaction can make it hard to breathe.

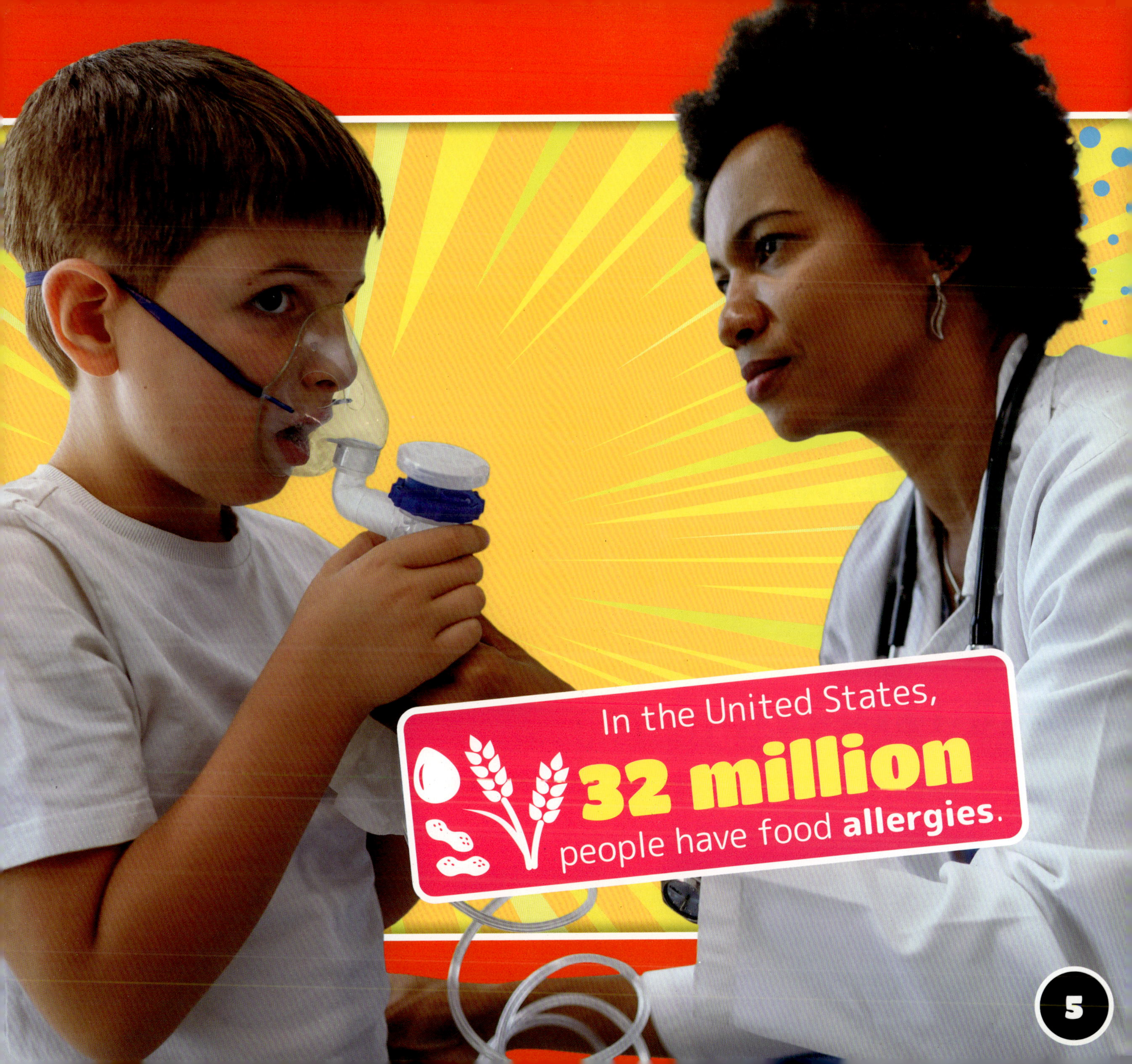

In the United States, **32 million** people have food **allergies**.

Signs and Symptoms

An allergic reaction can cause an itchy rash or sneezing.

It can also make the throat feel tight.

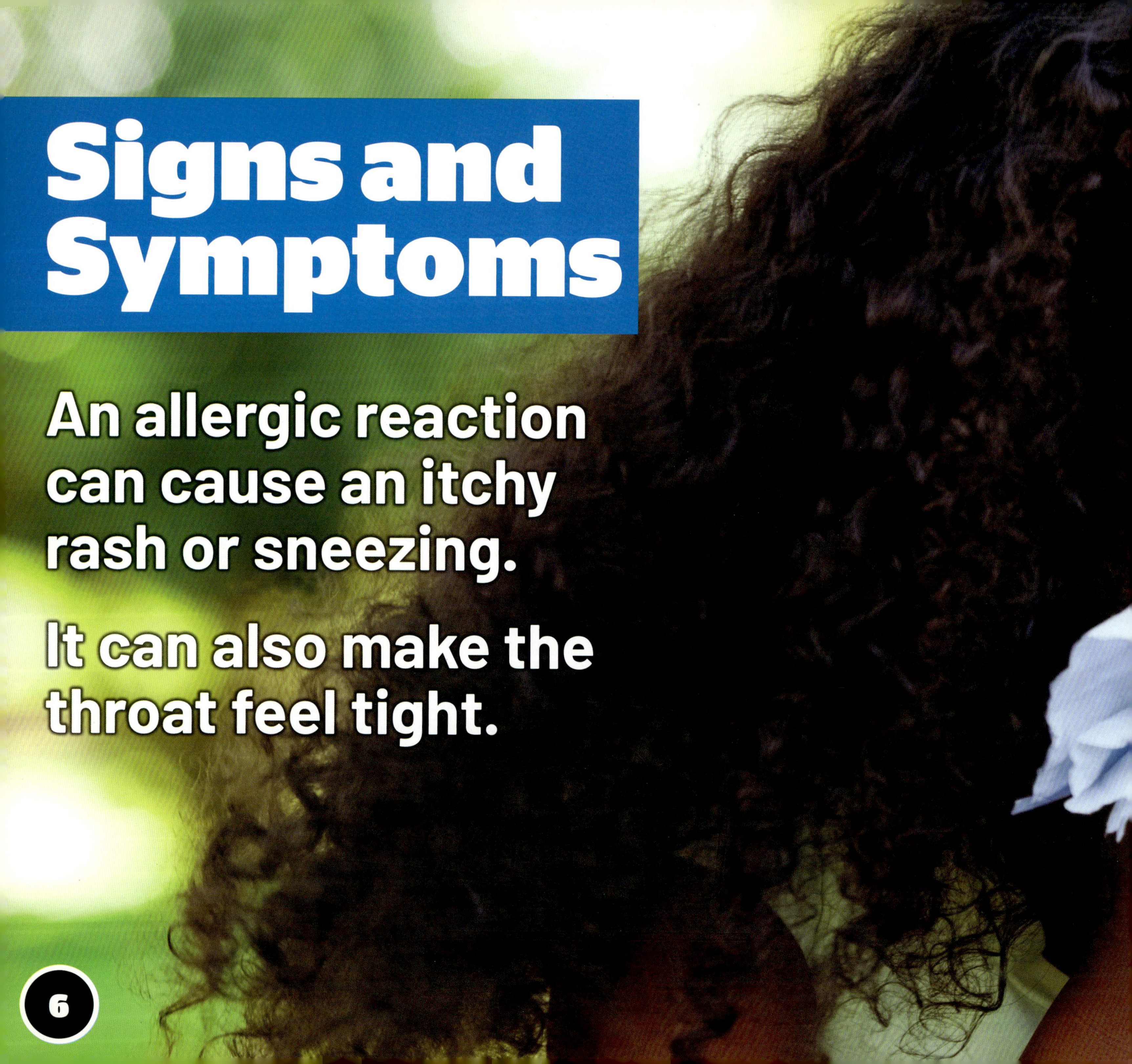

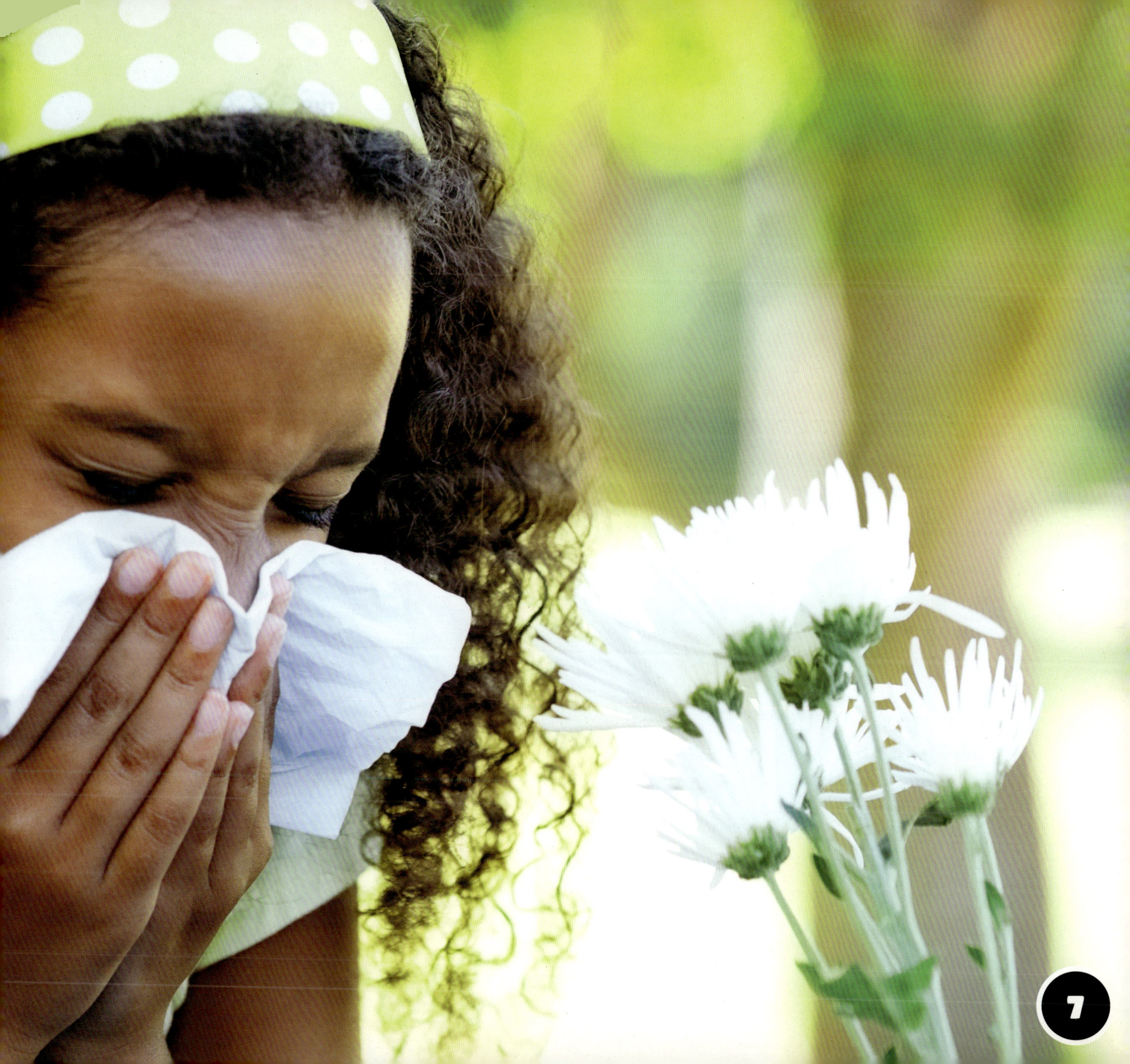

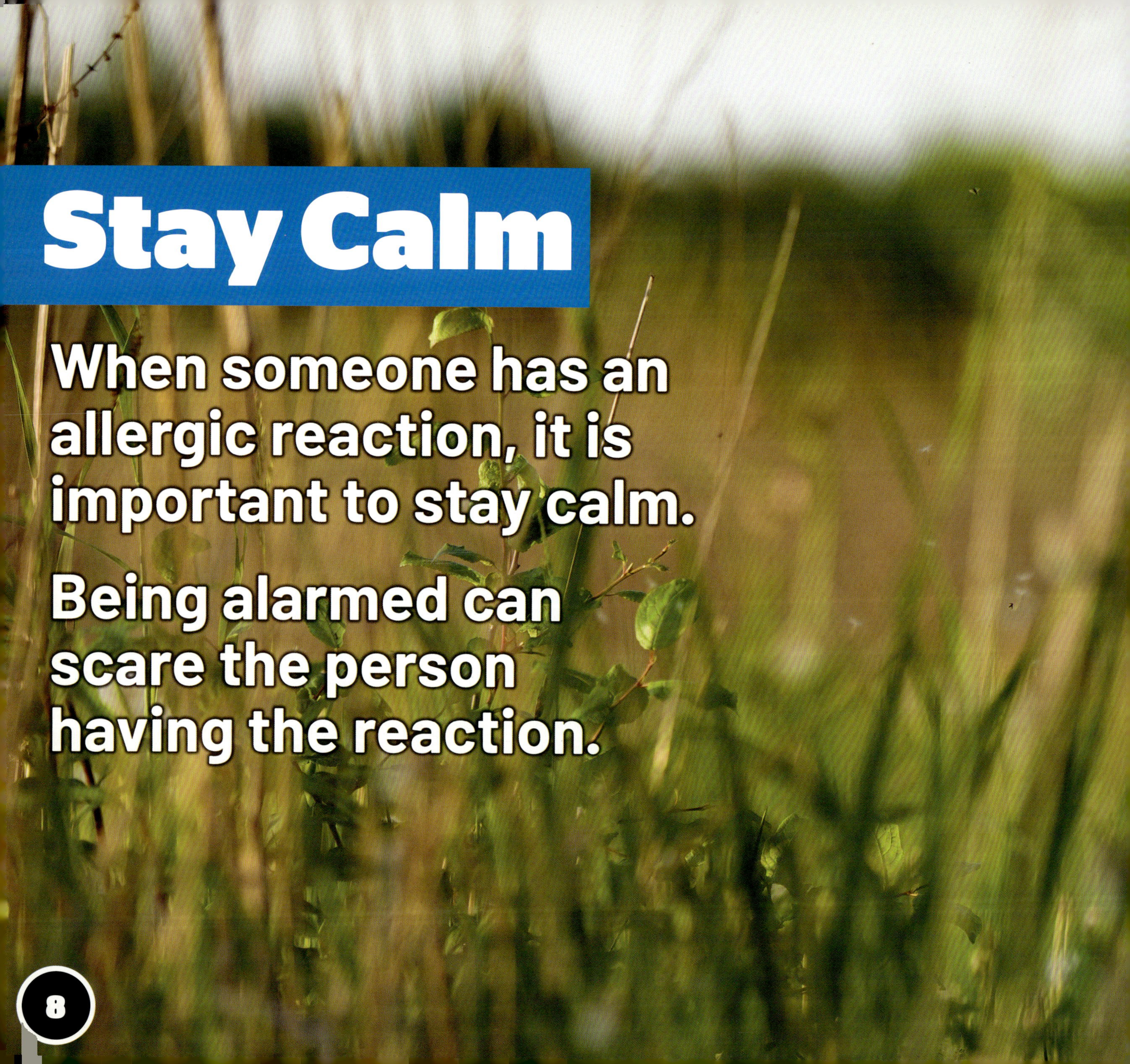

Stay Calm

When someone has an allergic reaction, it is important to stay calm.

Being alarmed can scare the person having the reaction.

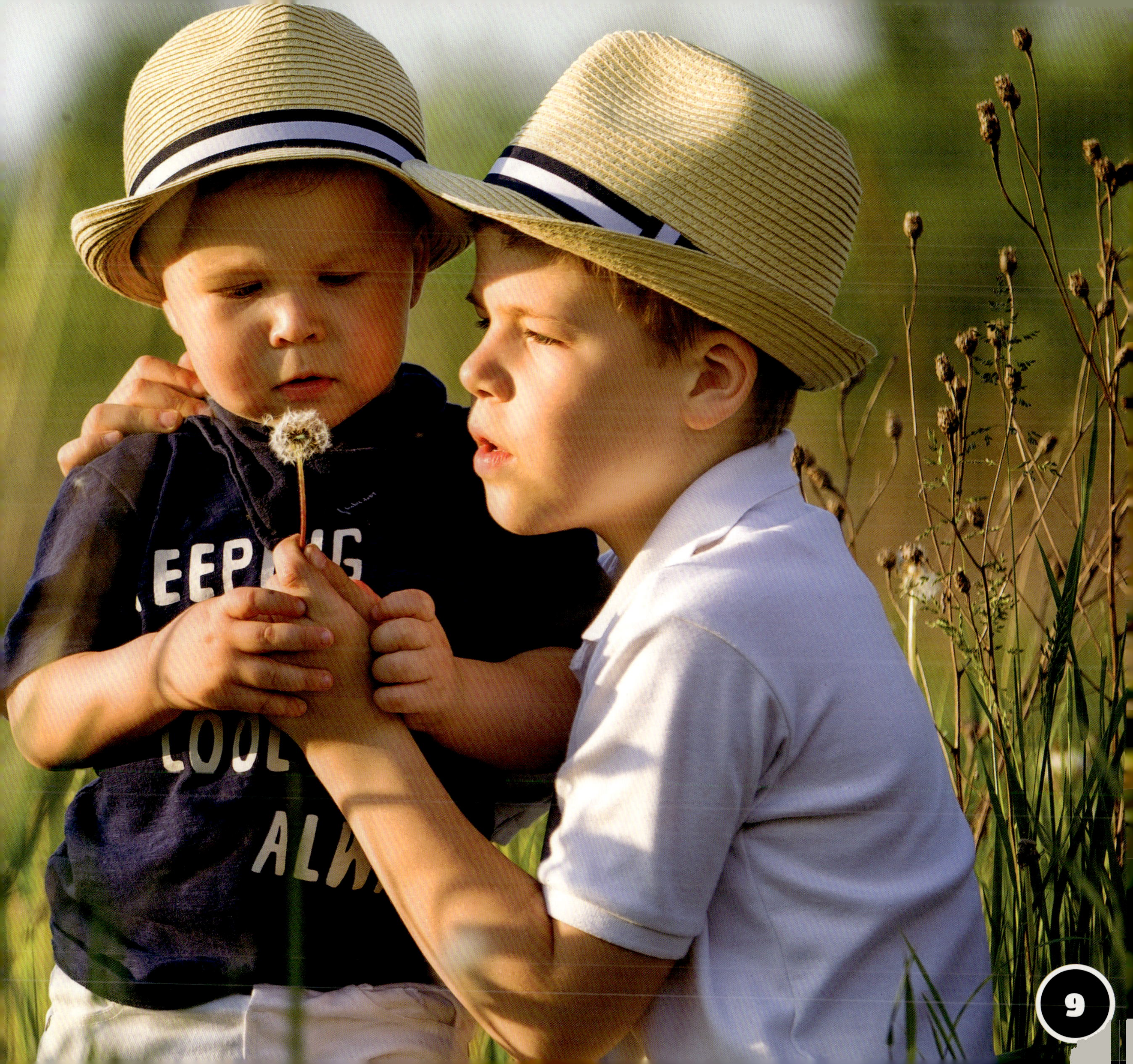

Call 9-1-1

Call 9-1-1 if the allergic reaction is really bad.

The 9-1-1 operator will need to know your name, where you are, and what the emergency is.

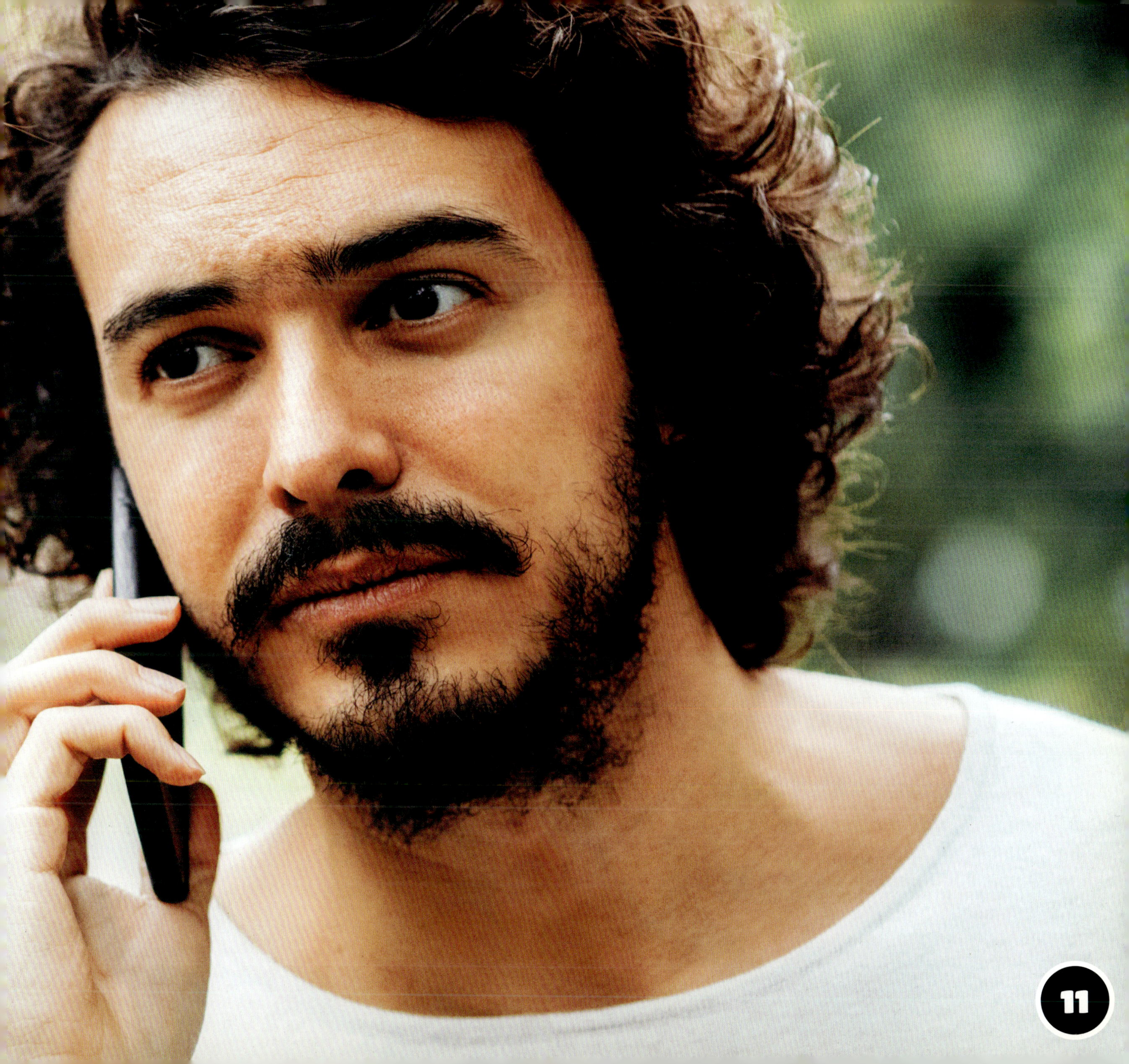

Move Away

Someone having an allergic reaction should move away from the cause.

The reaction will not start to get better until the cause is far away.

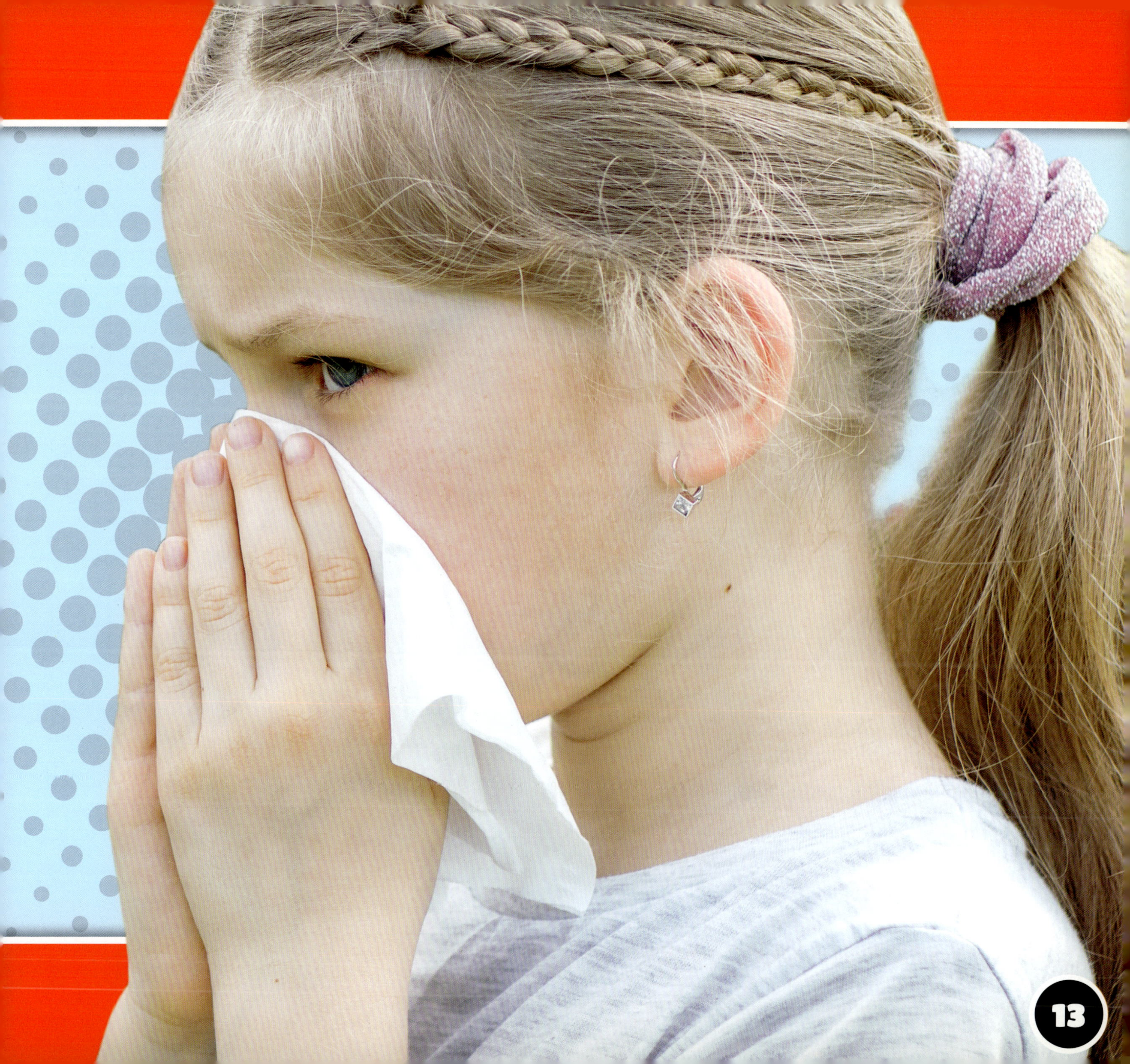

Give Medicine

A person with an allergy may have medicine for it.

Some medicines make itching go away. Others help people to breathe.

Someone having an allergic reaction may need help with his or her medicine.

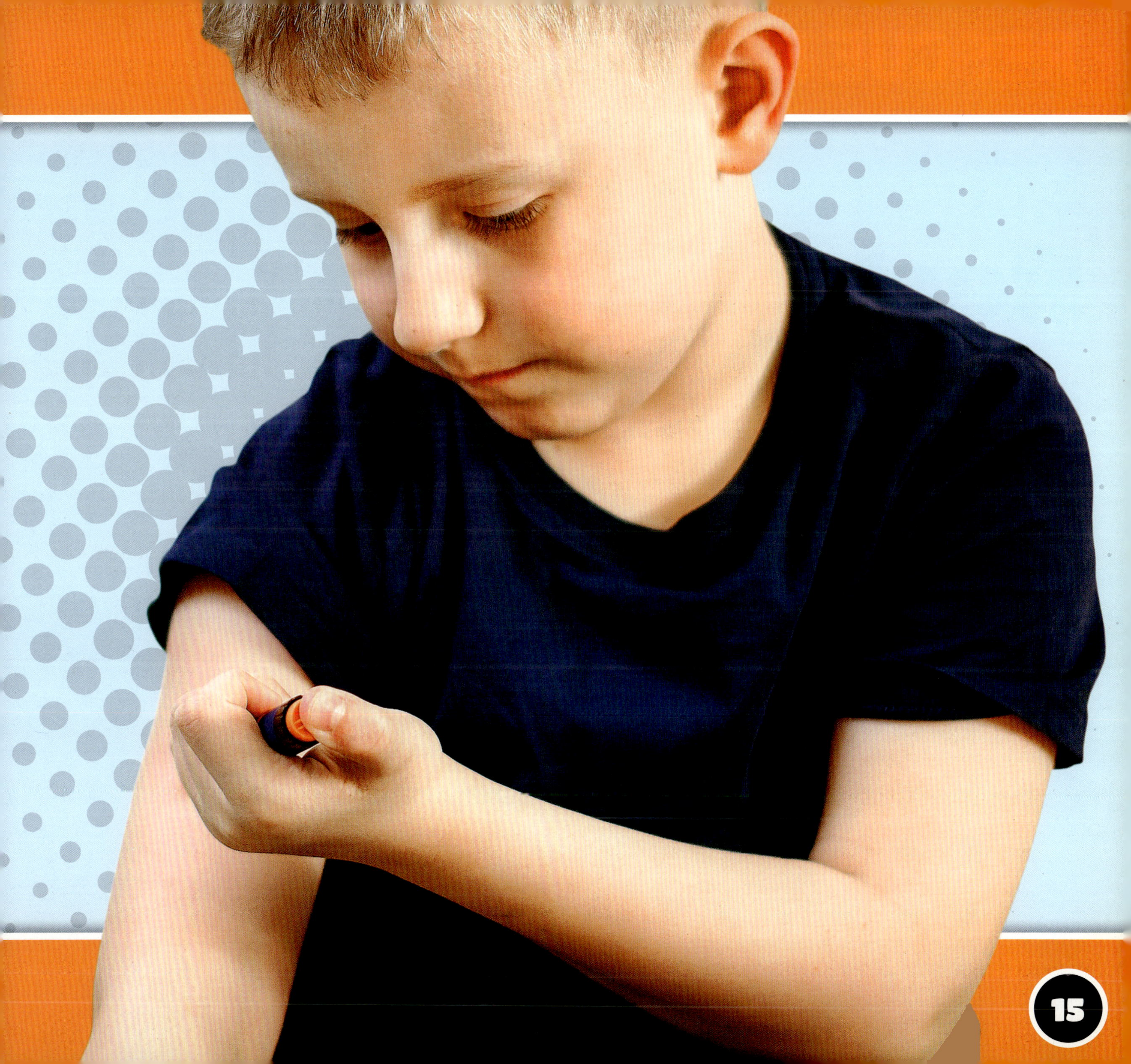

Rest

Medicine needs
time to work.

A person should sit down
and breathe slowly while
the reaction goes away.

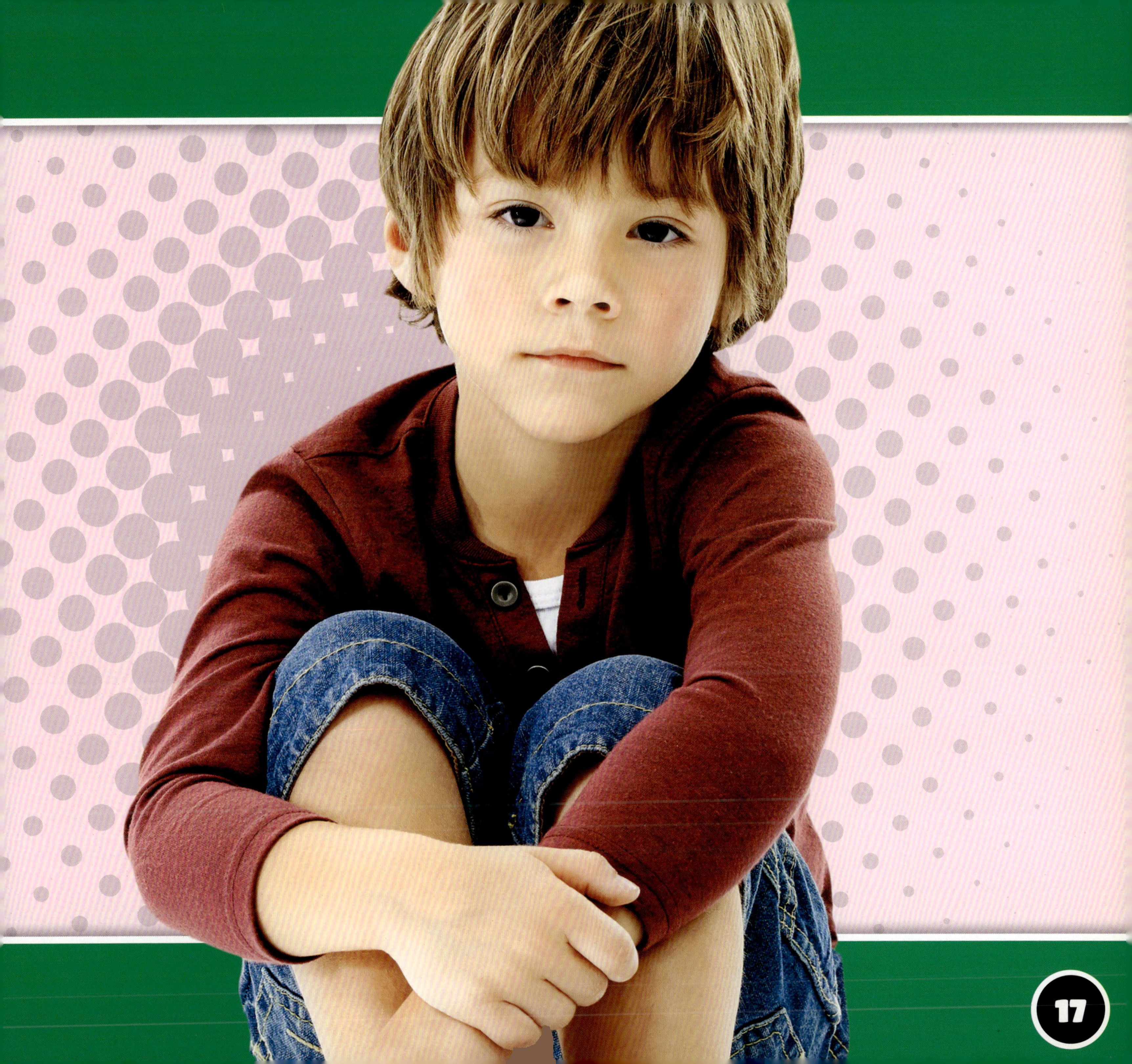

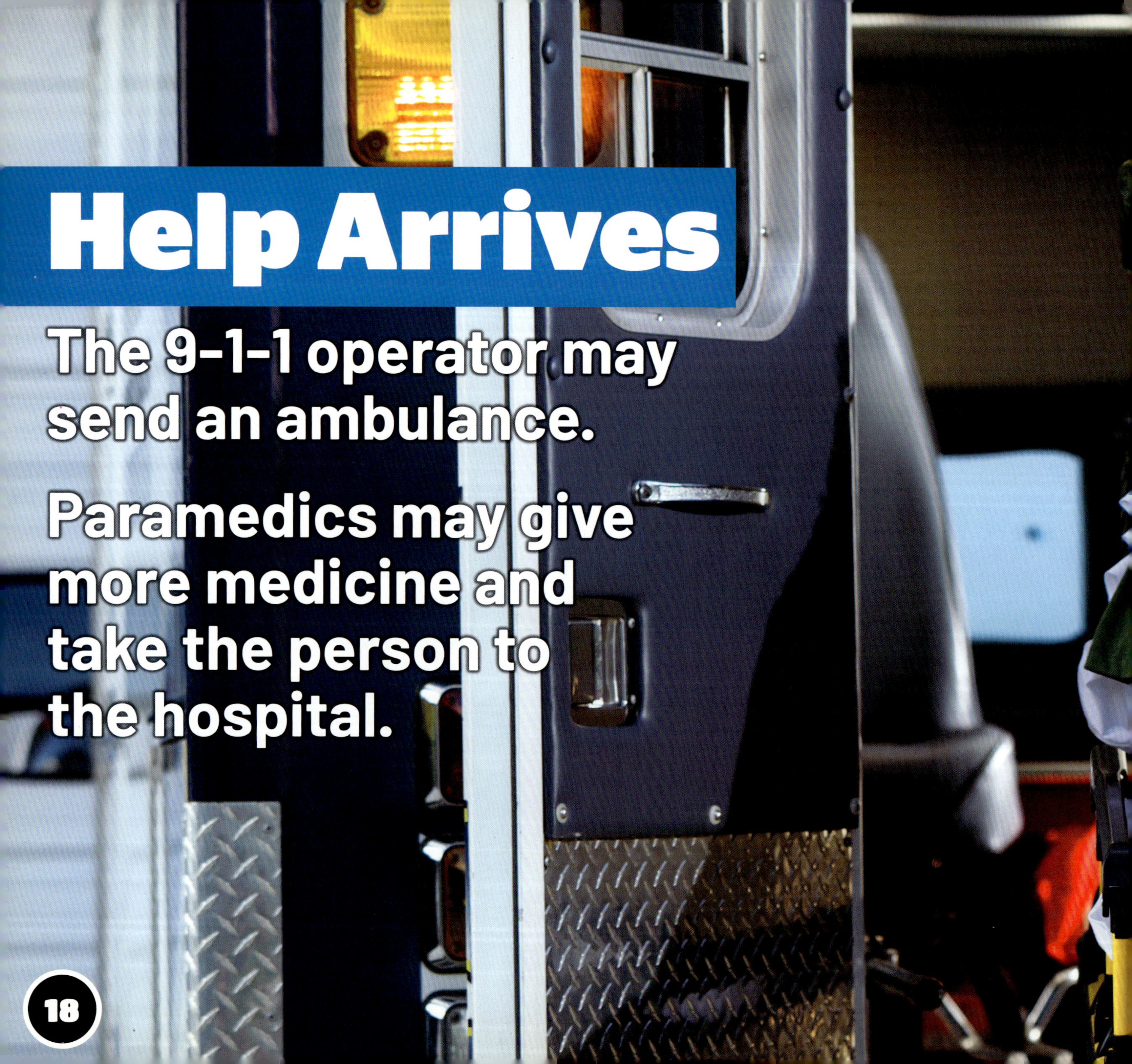

Help Arrives

The 9-1-1 operator may send an ambulance.

Paramedics may give more medicine and take the person to the hospital.

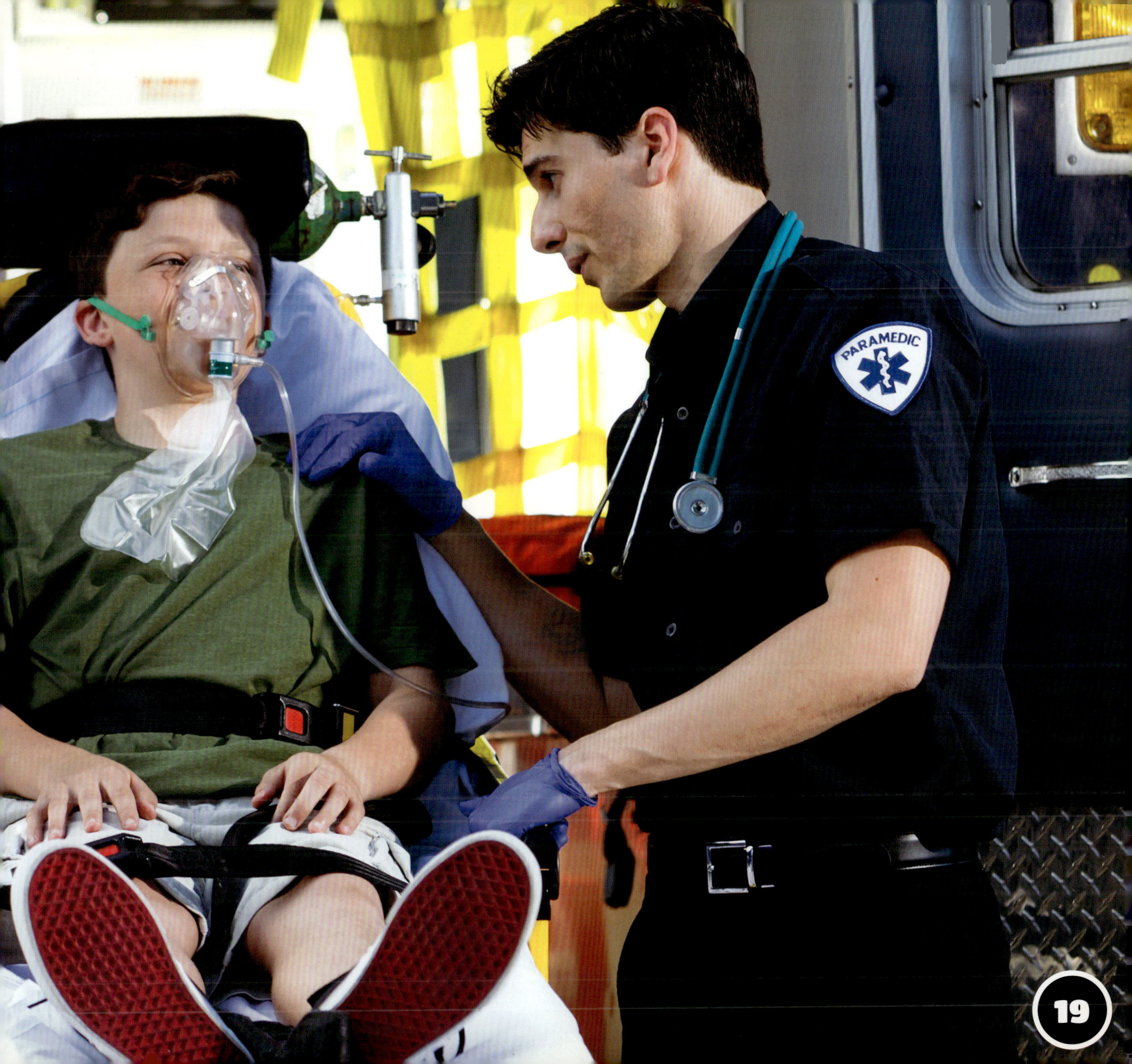
PARAMEDIC

Preventative Measures

People with allergies should try to stay away from things they are allergic to.

They should always carry their allergy medicine with them.

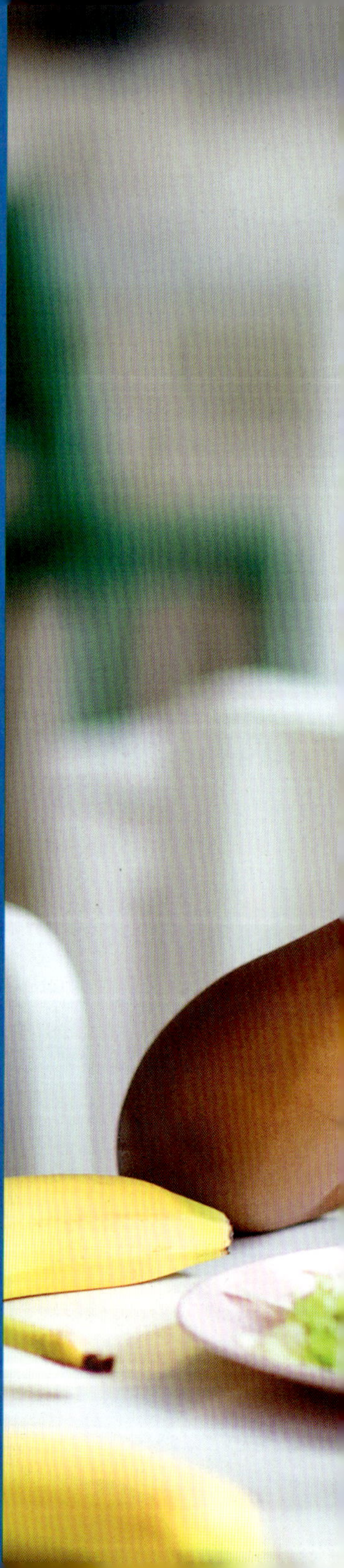

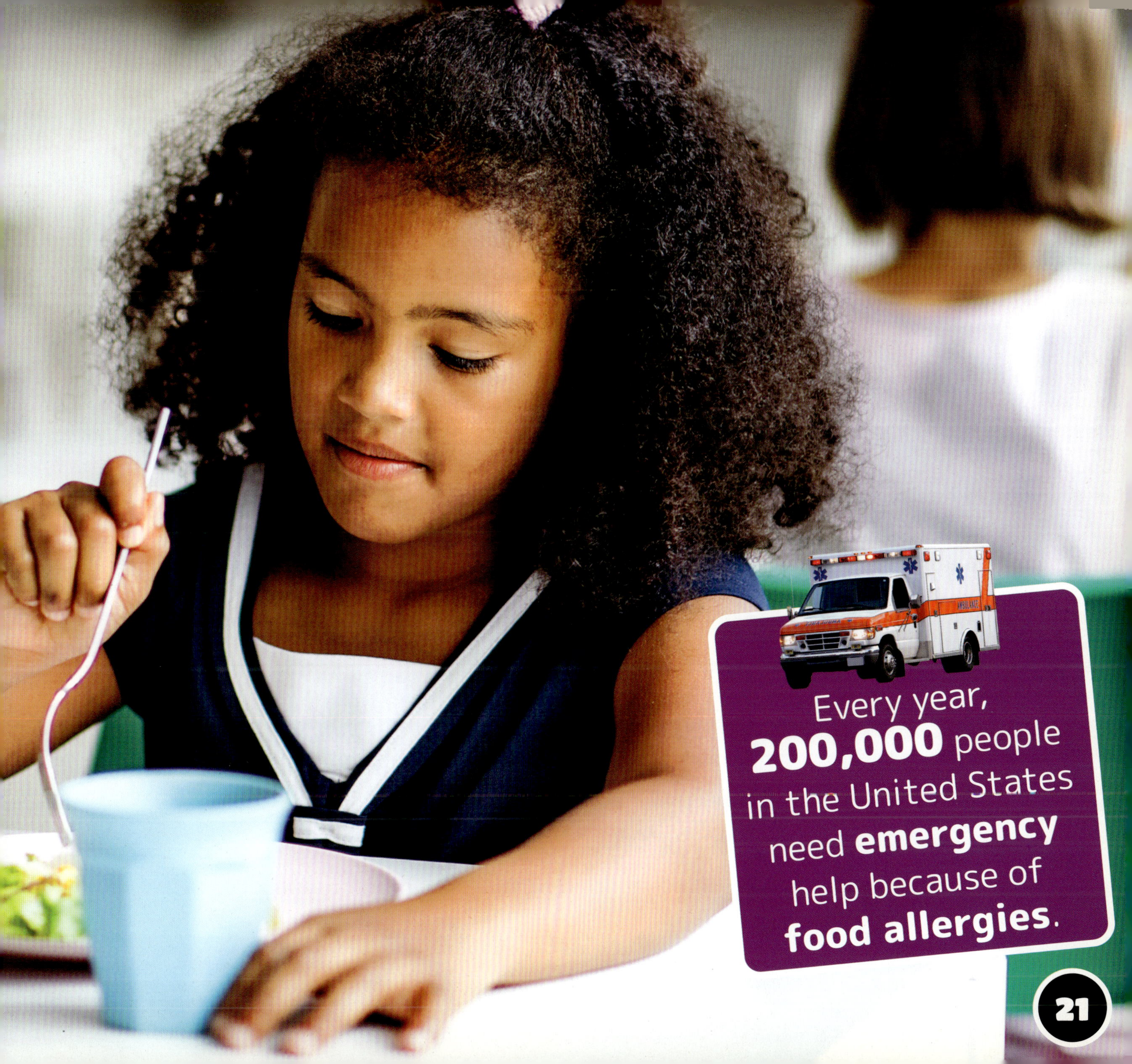

Every year, **200,000** people in the United States need **emergency** help because of **food allergies**.

EMERGENCY PROCEDURES

These pages provide detailed information that expands on the emergency found in the book. They are intended to be used by adults as a learning support to help young readers understand the correct responses to each emergency featured in the *In Case of Emergency* series.

Pages 4–5

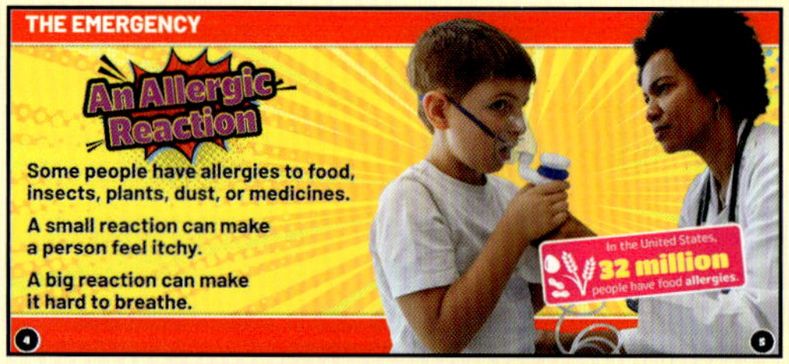

Some people have allergies to food, insects, plants, dust, or medicines. An allergy is a response to a substance that a person is sensitive to. Responses can be mild or severe. An allergic reaction can cause a person's airway to narrow. This makes breathing difficult. Allergens such as insect bites, foods, medications, animals, or pollen can trigger allergic reactions. There are no cures for allergies, but the symptoms can be managed.

Pages 6–7

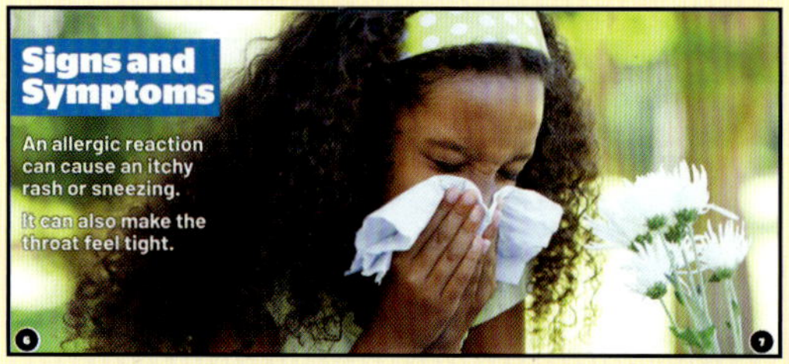

An allergic reaction can cause an itchy rash or sneezing. Symptoms of an allergic reaction include rashes, itchiness, sneezing, swelling in the mouth and throat, and trouble breathing. Someone suffering from an allergic reaction may also become anxious or panic as he or she struggles to breathe.

Pages 8–9

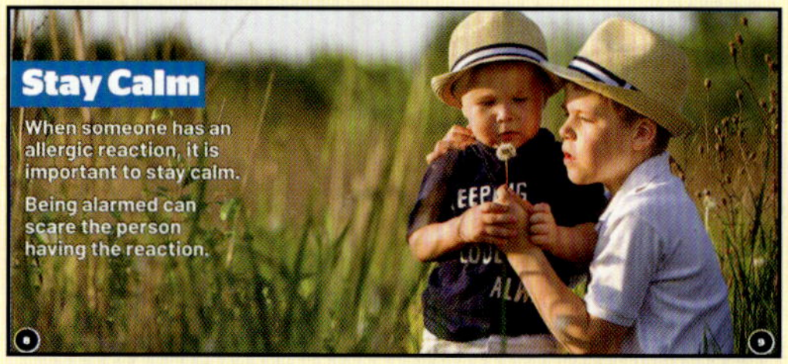

When someone has an allergic reaction, it is important to stay calm. It is important to stay calm during any emergency. It is especially important for the person experiencing an allergic reaction to remain calm. If a person having a severe reaction starts to panic, he or she will have a hard time breathing, tightening the airways even further. The person assisting someone having an allergic reaction should remain calm. This helps to keep the patient calm, too. It also helps the person to make good, measured decisions about what to do.

Pages 10–11

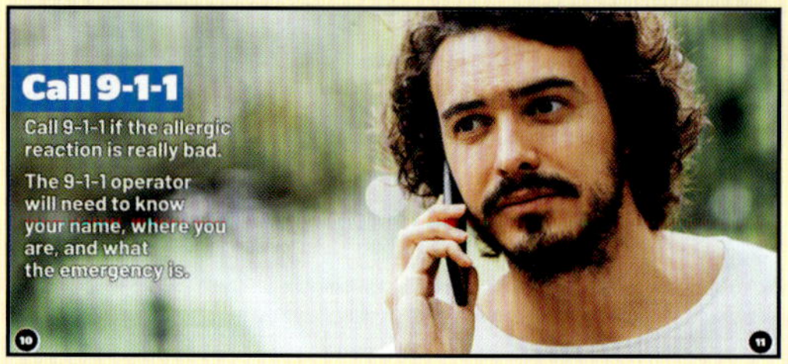

Call 9-1-1 if the allergic reaction is really bad. A call to 9-1-1 should only be placed in emergency situations. Not all allergic reactions are severe enough to warrant calling 9-1-1. Call 9-1-1 if a person having an allergic reaction has trouble breathing. Even if the person experiencing an allergic reaction has applied an EpiPen, seek emergency help. In less severe cases, an allergic reaction can be treated without the assistance of emergency medical services (EMS) or a doctor.

Pages 12–13

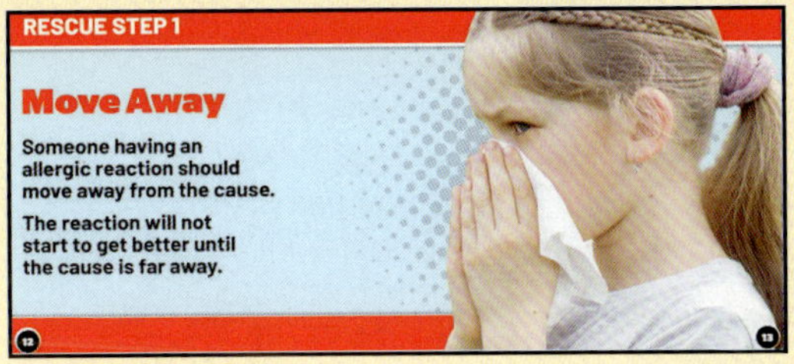

Someone having an allergic reaction should move away from the cause. The first step in treating an allergic reaction is to remove the patient from the allergen causing it. Any treatment of a reaction, especially if it is a severe reaction, may be ineffective if the allergen is still able to affect the person.

Pages 14–15

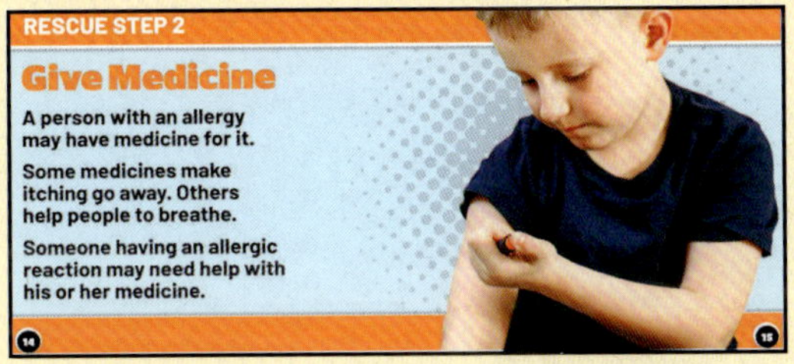

A person with an allergy may have medicine for it. Mild allergic reactions may be treatable with over-the-counter medications. A person with a severe allergy may carry an EpiPen. It is important that the proper medication be administered as quickly as possible in order to minimize the severity of the allergic reaction.

Pages 16–17

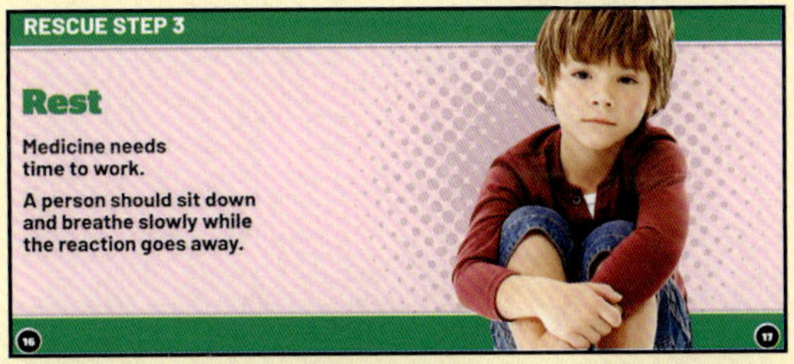

Medicine needs time to work. It is important to let the body recover after an allergic reaction. For severe reactions, the person should go to a hospital or other emergency medical center. He or she will need to be monitored. Even if the symptoms of the reaction seem to be going away, there is a chance the reaction could flare back up as medications wear off.

Pages 18–19

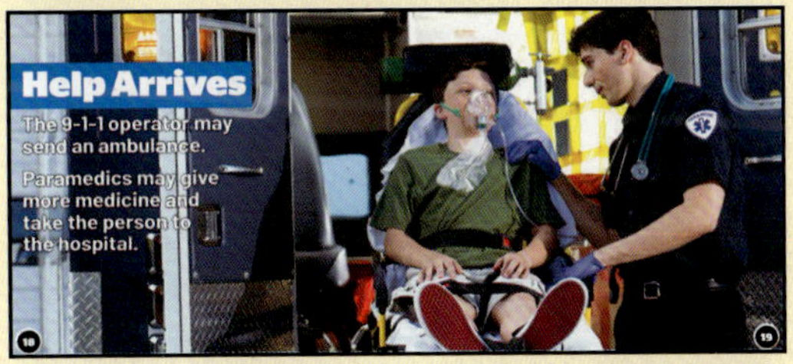

The 9-1-1 operator may send an ambulance. If paramedics have been sent by 9-1-1, they will assess the situation and monitor the person having an allergic reaction. Paramedics are trained to administer medicines that will help relax the person's airway and make breathing easier. Even if the reaction seems to be over, paramedics may still take the person to the hospital so he or she can be monitored and evaluated by a doctor.

Pages 20–21

People with allergies should try to stay away from things they are allergic to. Since there is no cure for allergic reactions, a person with a known allergy must try to avoid coming in contact with the things that trigger his or her allergies. If a doctor prescribes an EpiPen, it is important to carry it at all times. It is also important to know how to use the EpiPen.

KEY WORDS

Research has shown that as much as 65 percent of all written material published in English is made up of 300 words. These 300 words cannot be taught using pictures or learned by sounding them out. They must be recognized by sight. This book contains 72 common sight words to help young readers improve their reading fluency and comprehension. This book also teaches young readers several important content words, such as proper nouns. These words are paired with pictures to aid in learning and improve understanding.

Page	Sight Words First Appearance
4	a, an, big, can, food, hard, have, it, make, or, people, plants, small, some, the, to
5	in, states
6	also, and
8	being, has, important, is, when
10	are, call, if, know, name, need, really, what, where, will, you, your
12	away, far, from, get, move, not, should, start, until
14	for, give, go, help, her, his, may, others, with
16	down, time, while, work
18	more, take
20	always, carry, their, them, they, things, try
21	because, every, of, year

Page	Content Words First Appearance
4	allergic reaction, allergies, dust, emergency, insects, medicines, person
5	United States
6	rash, signs, symptoms, throat
10	operator
12	cause, step
18	ambulance, hospital, paramedics
20	preventative measures

Published by AV2
14 Penn Plaza 9th Floor New York, NY 10122
Website: www.av2books.com

Library of Congress Cataloging-in-Publication Data

Names: Friesen, Helen Lepp, 1961- author. | Smith, Ryan, author.
Title: Allergies / Helen Lepp Friesen and Ryan Smith.
Description: New York, NY : AV2, [2021] | Series: In case of emergency | Audience: Ages 5-9 | Audience: Grades 2-3
Identifiers: LCCN 2020014486 (print) | LCCN 2020014487 (ebook) | ISBN 9781791126568 (library binding) | ISBN 9781791126575 (paperback) | ISBN 9781791126582 | ISBN 9781791126599
Subjects: LCSH: Allergy--Juvenile literature. | Medical emergencies--Juvenile literature.
Classification: LCC RC584 .F75 2021 (print) | LCC RC584 (ebook) | DDC 616.97/3--dc23
LC record available at https://lccn.loc.gov/2020014486
LC ebook record available at https://lccn.loc.gov/2020014487

Printed in Guangzhou, China
1 2 3 4 5 6 7 8 9 0 24 23 22 21 20

052020
100919

Project Coordinator: Ryan Smith
Art Director: Terry Paulhus

The publisher acknowledges iStock and Shutterstock as its primary image suppliers for this title.